Overcoming
Senior Moments:

Vanishing Thoughts—Causes and Remedies.

By **Frances Meiser**
and
Nina Anderson

Designed and Illustrated by Yvonne Cecile Bossard

Overcoming
Senior Moments:

Vanishing Thoughts—Causes and Remedies.

ISBN: 0-9701110-9-6
Library of Congress Catalog Card Number 00-136421

Printed in Canada

The concepts, techniques and methods discussed in **Overcoming Senior Moments**, are not intended as medical advice, but as suggested *complementary therapeutic regimens* to be considered only if deemed adequate by both patients and their chosen health professionals.

New Century Publishing 2000

Canada	United States
60 Bullock Dr., Unit 6	P.O. Box 36
Markham, ON L3P 3P2	E. Canaan, CT 05024
905.471.5711	860.824.5301

Cover Design: Janine White
Cover photo: Digital Imagery © 2001 Photodisc, Inc.

To my Uncle Jack.
And to all the other families
who lost a loved one too early
due to brain dementia.
Plus, to all the wonderful
people who came along
to help me shed some light
on these problems—
Thanks for caring
and sharing.

—Frances Meiser

Overcoming Senior Moments:
Vanishing Thoughts—The Causes and the Remedies.

continues next page . . .

Meet "S-naps" the brainy neuron. Throughout this book S-naps will provide interesting asides and tidbits of information.

Contents

Contents continues . . .

Chapter 4

"There is a vitality, a life force, an energy, a quickening, that is translated through you into action, and there is only one of you in all time, this expression is unique, and if you block it, it will never exist through any other medium and will be lost."

—Martha Graham,

1894–1991

The Problem

It really doesn't matter whether your age is six or sixty, we all have memory lapses from time to time. We used to think that when we reached retirement age, we were expected to repeat ourselves, and to forget to turn off the stove. Unfortunately, this behavior is showing up at earlier ages; from simply forgetting where you put your keys, to looking at a familiar friend and not remembering her name.

Memory loss may be attributed to the following:

> Aging
> Alcohol overuse
> Aluminum toxicity
> Alzheimer's
> Anesthetics
> Chemical synthesis inadequacies
> Chronic infections
> Depression
> Drugs
> "Bad" fats
> Head trauma
> Menopause
> Mineral deficiencies
> Oxidative damage to the brain which effect nerve's
>   myelin sheath
> Seizures
> Stroke
> Synthetic estrogens
> Table sugar
> Vitamin deficiencies

The worst form of memory loss is Alzheimer's disease. First discovered in 1906, Alzheimer's has grown to be the fourth leading cause of death for adults. It affects six million people and costs 100 billion dollars a year. It is showing up in young people as well as the elderly.

A normal brain is composed of tissue that is plump and healthy with tight spaces between the tissues. A brain suffering from Alzheimer's is shriveled, and the tissues have large gaps between them as a result of nerve cells dying. When enough nerve cells die, memory is affected. Amyloid plaque, which kills brain cells, may form when deficiencies of melatonin (a hormone produced in the brain) exist. This was normally considered a condition of aging. Unfortunately, similar states are appearing in younger people, where chemical imbalances exist that throw off hormone function.

More reasons for brain atrophy.

Neurons communicate with each other through structures called synapses, which release a transmitter chemical. If these chemicals are either deficient or excessive, brain function will be impaired.

Brain regulators.

Acetylcholine affects memory, serotonin regulates mood, noradrenaline influences mood and autonomic function, and dopamine affects motor coordination. These regulators may be upset if the body's normal chemistry is altered through lack of specific nutrients, vitamins, minerals, or through emotional stressors. They can create imbalances in the brain, and reduce the amount of information transmitted from cell to cell.

The symptoms of Attention Deficit Disorder are thought to be related to a brain chemical imbalance; primarily, serotonin. Serotonin is manufactured in the brain in the presence of Vitamin B_6 and an essential amino acid, tryptophan, which is supplied by protein. When deficiencies of serotonin exist, neurotransmitter signals are compromised and behavioral anomalies surface. An overabundance of insulin also reduces serotonin levels, and induces foggy thinking, by reducing blood sugar levels to the brain. Magnesium must be present in the body in sufficient quantity to regulate this overabundance of insulin. Many children diagnosed with A.D.D. have low magnesium at the cellular level.[1]

Side effects of prescription drugs can also affect brain function. If you experience memory loss while taking drugs, you should mention it to your physician. At times, forgetful behavior

[1]Bell, Rachel, Peiper, H., *The A.D.D. and A.D.H.D. Diet!*, Safe Goods, 1997.

may be associated with a drug. If this type of senior moment is further misdiagnosed drug protocols for preventing Alzheimer's or Dementia may be prescribed when all you may need to do is stop taking the drug.

Common drugs that may affect memory are:

Aldomet	Mellaril
Ascendin	Miltown
Dalmane	Pepcid
Elavil	Symmetrel
Equanil	Tagamet
Haldol	Valium
Inderal	Zantac

Anxiety, depression and stress.

Other unseen culprits may also affect your memory. Since brain function is primarily chemical in nature, it is logical to assume that emotions affecting our body-chemistry also affect neural function. Anxiety, depression and stress are the most common emotions that can have a negative effect on chemical-dependent neurotransmitter function. Distraction, fatigue, apathy, loss of sensory perception (vision, hearing) and too much information to process (neural overload), all may induce temporary memory loss.

A strong factor in brain function is the ability of our body to operate as it is designed to do. Since the brain is mostly water, it is common sense to assume that we must stay hydrated. Specific nutrients play a constructive part in nerve health, and therefore, if we have dietary deficiencies, memory loss may surface.

Brain health basics.

Our environment also plays a big part in the health of our brain. Toxic or chemical-laden indoor air, highly chlorinated un-filtered water, pesticide ingestion, mold, exposure to electromag-netic fields and certain food additives all can compromise our immune system. Animals used for food are many times fed hormone-laden feed to fatten them up. Synthetic estrogen hormones may remain in animal tissue after slaughter and end up in your meat. In some cases, Alzheimer's has been linked to these synthetic estrogens. Most food additives and environmental toxins lead to alterations in normal bodily operation, that can then stress the chemical balance of the brain. Basics that need to be addressed as absolutes for brain health are depicted in the next chapter.

Supplemental help.

By following these recommendations your memory may be restored. However, if you have not been supporting your immune system, you may require additional help. For supplements that can act as treatments for memory loss, refer to Chapter Four.

"Whew—that's a heap of info!

Here's a look from a playful, visual perspective for your right brain to enjoy!

The Basic Remedy

This is a Diesel Engine.

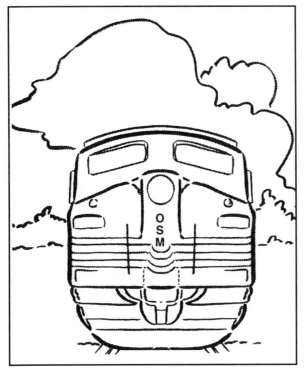

To keep a diesel running at full speed
you need to fuel, oil and maintain it daily.

The Basic Remedy

Your Brain
is <u>YOUR</u> engine.

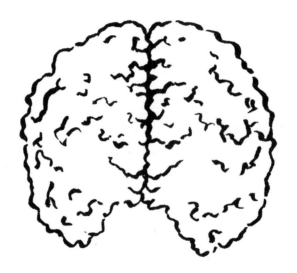

To keep your engine running at full speed
you need to
feed, water and exercise it daily.

Your brain consists of about:

75% water,

10% fat and

8% protein.

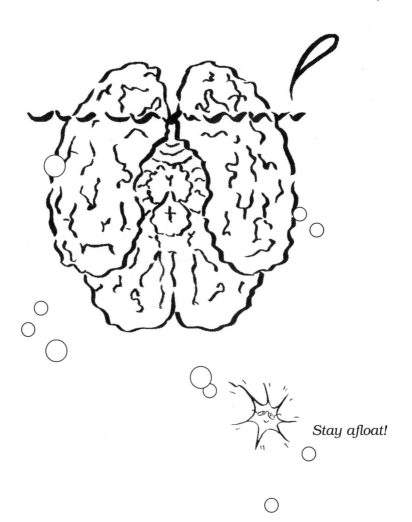

Stay afloat!

Good brain care starts with

plain water!

Cool, clean water.

Water is the conductor
needed for electrical impulses to carry information
when thoughts occur.

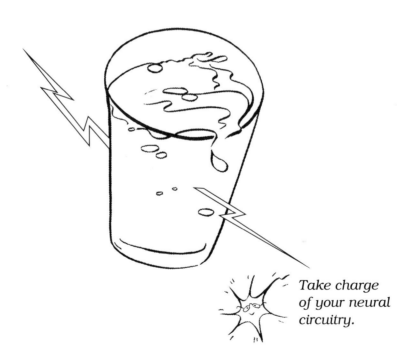

*Take charge
of your neural
circuitry.*

Your brain needs 8 to 12

~~buckets~~

big glasses

of clean water each day!

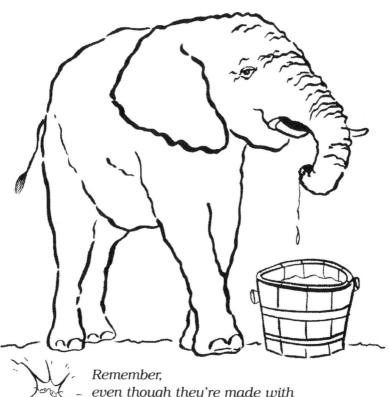

Remember,
even though they're made with
water—coffee, tea, etc. **don't count!**

Since your brain is composed of

75% water,

you need to fill it up daily for maximum brain function.
Your engine cannot attain peak performance
if it is dehydrated.

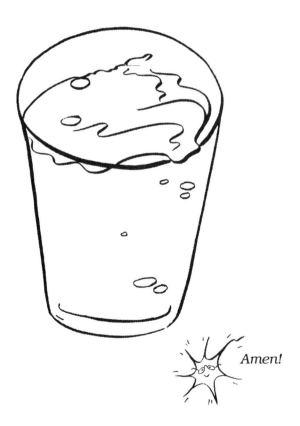

Amen!

Drink filtered water instead of tap water.

Chemicals and
pesticides are trapped by
running tap water through a

FILTER.

But Note: Filtering also traps *beneficial minerals*
which are important to your brain.
After filtering you must add them back in.

*By the way:
We'll give you more
information on water filters
and how to add minerals later.*

Have you experienced
a vanishing thought
called . . .

. . . A Senior Moment?

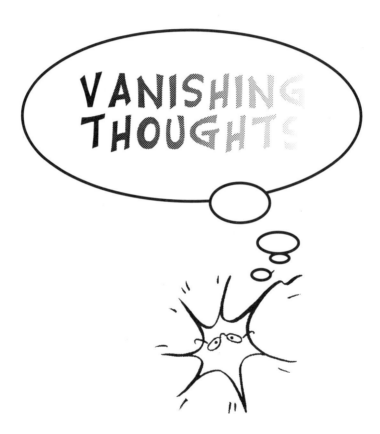

*Drink plenty of clean, filtered
water so electrical brain impulses
can flow where they need to go!*

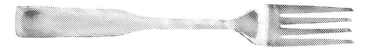

Brain Food.

Nourish your Brain!
Your diet affects your cognitive function.
Decreased attention and loss of concentration
are among the first signs of nutritional deprivation.

By the way:
Specific brain nutrition
preserves neural pathways
for the future.

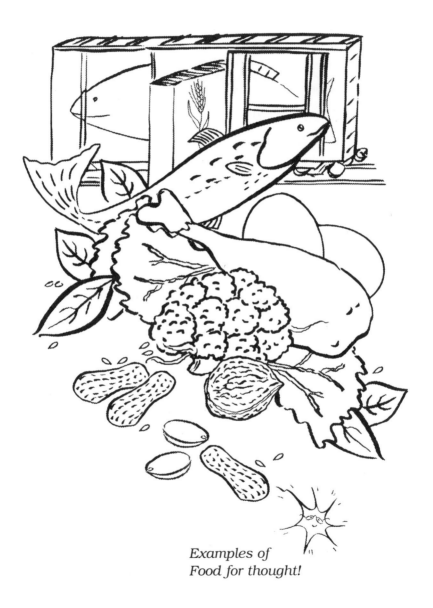

*Examples of
Food for thought!*

Brain foods are:

Nuts,

like walnuts and peanuts.

Whole grains

of rye, millet, brown rice,
oats, whole wheat and wheat germ.
But *not* white rice or white bread.

Protein foods,

such as seeds, lentils,
broccoli, eggs, sprouted soy,
powdered greens like spirulina,
sunflower sprouts,
tuna, salmon, sardines
and *lean* meats. For example, turkey,

and

Flax.

Flax seed oil comes from hard, shiny, golden brown seed that looks like tiny birdseed.

To be of greatest benefit to your brain, the seeds must be ground and extremely fresh.

The natural seed is tasty when spooned on cereal, put into pancakes or muffins or sprinkled atop yogurt. You may also obtain the oil in capsule form which may be taken as a supplement.

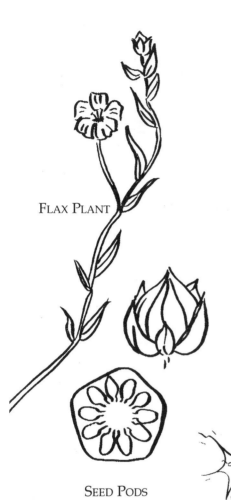

FLAX PLANT

SEED PODS

Check resources at the back of this book for more details on Flax Seed Oil and other "good" fats.

Why Flax?

Flax seed oil helps protect
the central information system in your brain.

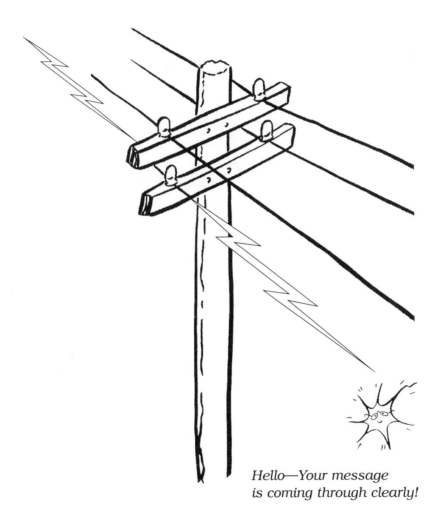

*Hello—Your message
is coming through clearly!*

The "good" fat in flax seeds makes a good,
strong, protective coating around nerve fibers
called the myelin sheath.

*This coating helps your brain work smarter—**Not** harder.*

Yes!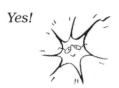

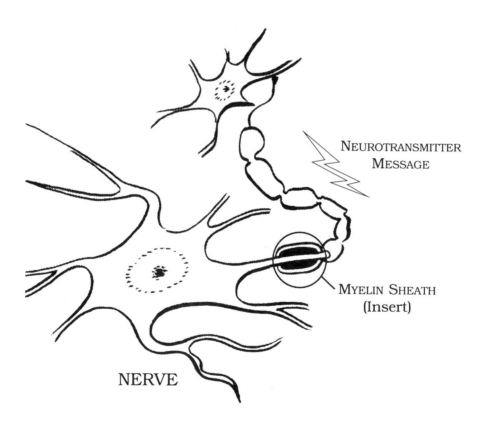

NEUROTRANSMITTER
MESSAGE

MYELIN SHEATH
(Insert)

NERVE

Also excellent for brain cell function
is the oil in salmon and tuna fish.

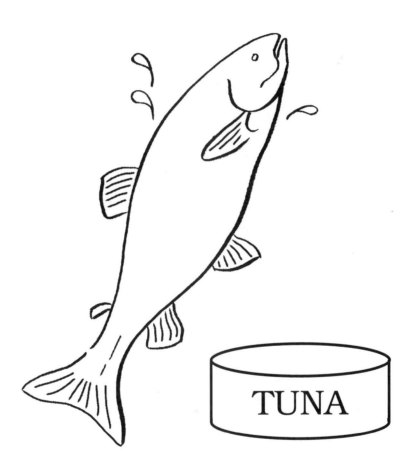

While we're on the subject of good foods—

The Acceptable Edible Egg . . . The Perfect Food.

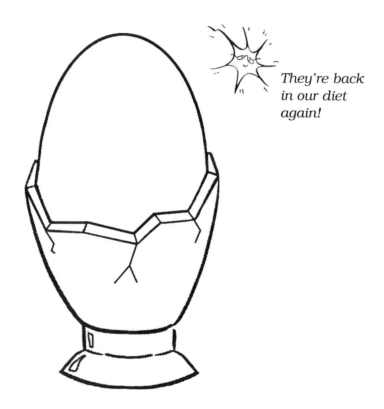

They're back
in our diet
again!

MOVEMENT!

In the beginning, as babies, we performed
suck, rollover and crawl movements.

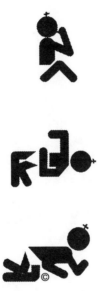

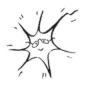 *Don't stop. Throughout our lives
we must continue to do them all!*

"Movement,
a natural process of life,
is now understood to be essential to learning,
creative thought and high level
formal reasoning."[2]

—Dr. Paul E. Dennison

Educational Kinesiologist and author of: *Brain Gym*©

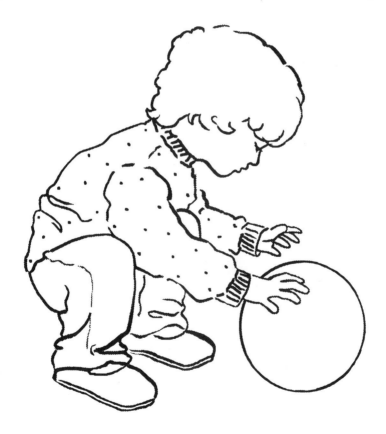

²Dennison, Dr. Paul E., Brain Gym, The Educational Kinesiology Foundation
800.356.2109 or www.braingym.org.

Circus strongman movements
do *not* help build a powerful brain.

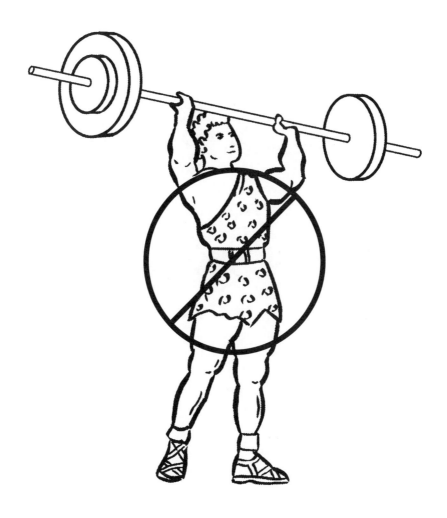

Movements that cross your midline are important!

Brain exercises, specifically gentle midline crossing movements, integrate right and left brain functions by creating new pathways for thinking and learning.

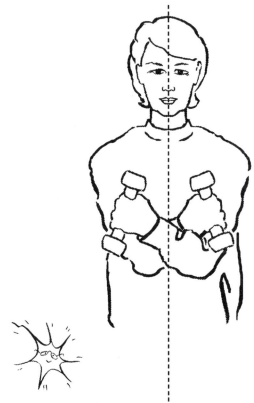

Your midline runs up and down your body through nose and navel.

As we do movements which cross our midline
the right and left sides of our brain begin to work together.

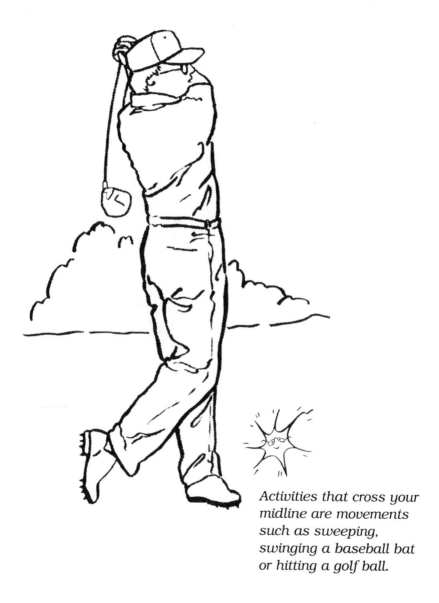

*Activities that cross your
midline are movements
such as sweeping,
swinging a baseball bat
or hitting a golf ball.*

. . . or other activities such as playing chess or music.

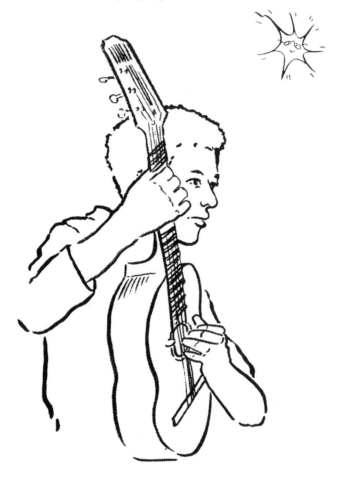

In addition to midline integration, music also stimulates "specific neuron connections in the abstract reasoning center of the brain and, in essence, makes subjects smarter."[3]

[3]Austin American Statesman, October 1998. Adapted from All–Mozart Music Diet Turns Lab Rats Into Maze Busters: Joseph B. Verrengia, A.P., October 4, 1998.

Exercising both sides of the brain
to get them working together is important because
the left brain sees only bits and pieces of the picture.

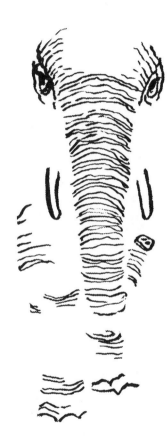

The right brain is the visual side.
It sees the complete picture.

Therefore, it is very important
to integrate both sides of your brain
with midline crossing movements.

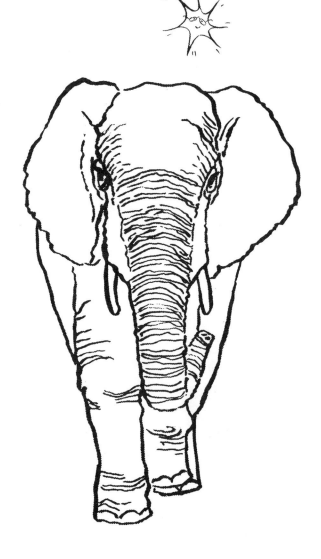

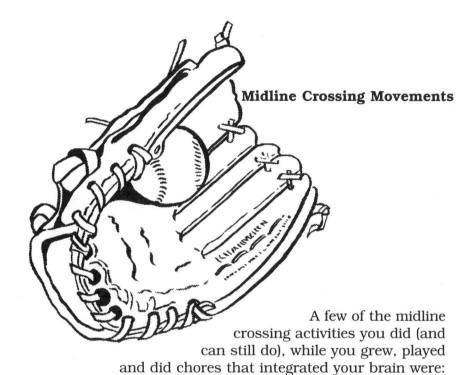

Midline Crossing Movements

A few of the midline crossing activities you did (and can still do), while you grew, played and did chores that integrated your brain were:

playing ping pong	dancing
playing jacks	doing cartwheels
playing badminton	playing the piano
jumping rope	sweeping
playing hop scotch	mopping
doing gymnastics	feather dusting
swimming	cutting out paper dolls
playing catch	finger painting
twirling a baton	marching in a band

participating in a drill team

drawing with sidewalk chalk

weeding

raking leaves

using a hand saw

ice skating

roller skating

playing baseball

playing softball

swinging a golf club

playing board games

shooting marbles

paddling a canoe

hitting a tetherball

dribbling a basketball

playing solitaire

performing magic tricks

shooting a hockey puck

playing touch football

twirling a baton

kicking a soccer ball

punching a boxing bag

doing puzzles

wrestling

twirling a hula-hoop

tossing a boomerang

skipping

yoga

Tai chi.

And as an adult you can explore:

Nia Technique—a blend of dance, martial arts and body integrating movements.

Through movement— Find your brilliance!

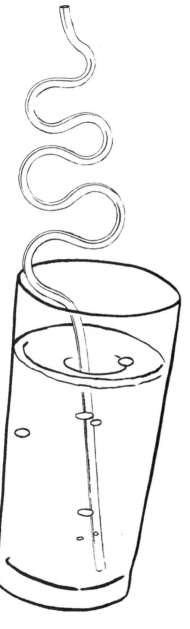

Remember suck, rollover and crawl? These activities helped our infant brains develop. One adult way to stimulate our brain is to sip eight to twelve ounces of liquid through a wiggle straw!

Sucking through "The crazy straw," according to The HANDLE Institute®, "stimulates both sides of the brain and, as such, enhances neural pathways. This provides many benefits including better eyesight, clearer speech and even bladder control."[4]

—Judith Bluestone

[4]Bluestone, Judith, The HANDLE Institute®, Seattle, WA.

How about rolling out of bed in the morning
and playing the piano.

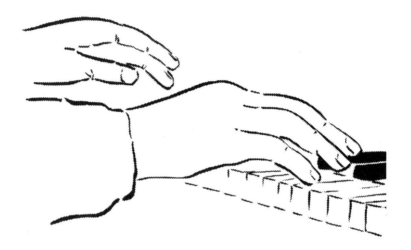

You may also do a slow, concentrated,
midline cross pattern crawl exercise while walking.

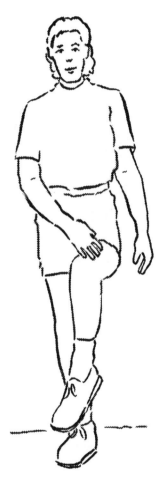

 Through movement—we find our brilliance.

Midline crossing movements
force the brain to make new routes—forge new trails.

Make home runs!
Take charge
of your neural circuitry.

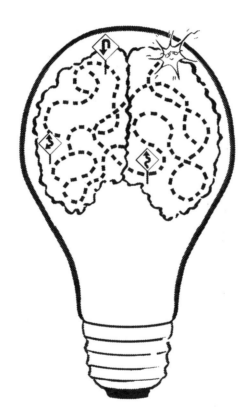

In whatever you do, find the fun part and

PLAY!

How you do a specific thing,
and what benefit you derive from it
can depend on whether
you think of it as work or

play.

*Play equals freedom and relaxation—
work equals constraint and responsibility,*

So go play!

The Basic Remedy

~y

The "nitty-gritty" about brain health

Water
Minerals
"Good" Fats
Enzymes
Brain Hazards
Exercise

WATER—A brain necessity.

The number one ingredient for brain health is so simple that most of us overlook it. *Water is life.* Since the brain is 75 percent water, it is logical to assume that a low water content will affect cognitive function. Many of us get busy and forget to drink water, or prefer something sweeter like carbonated drinks or juice or a hot drink, like tea or coffee. Although these substitutes do contain water, they are also considered food because of ingredients that need to be digested. This means that not all of the water goes to places in the body where it is needed.

Staying hydrated is essential for the health of the body. Athletes know this. Manufacturers have targeted them with so many different brands of bottled water that they may have difficulty choosing a favorite.

What Is and Is Not in Your Water?

When we say, "drink plenty of water," we caution you to consider water quality. Spring water can be the purist source of natural water, but very few of us live near an uncontaminated mountain brook. If you live in a city, chances are very likely your city water system has been treated with chlorine to kill bacteria. Unfortunately, when chlorine meets decaying plant matter, like that in your intestines, it can form trihalomethanes, which are known to cause cancer. Fluoride is also added to city water. In small quantities it helps protect teeth, but too much can actually cause mottling of the teeth.

If your tap water comes from a city water system, it is important that you consider purchasing a water filter. Countertop models are convenient and can do a great job of filtering out harmful additives. Bottled water is better than unfiltered tap water, but if kept for a long time (as in the store), it can actually grow bacteria. Well water is okay as long as you have it tested once in awhile for bacteria and heavy metals.

What is Missing from Most Water Sources?
MINERALS—The spark that helps you think.

Most of the water we get for drinking today is deficient in trace minerals. Unless it is from a virgin mountain stream, chances are that the water has lost its minerals on its trip from the reservoir to your tap. Since purified bottled water and filtered tap water have many of the essential trace minerals removed, it is necessary to add them back through supplementation.

Minerals are best added to your water by using a supplement that contains ionic minerals (the smallest form) in a liquid solution that delivers maximum absorption. Larger colloidal forms of mineral supplements (most available in pill form), are usually too large to squeeze into your cells and should therefore be your last choice.

Minerals that are attached to a carrier (example: calcium carbonate) are not elemental minerals. Carrier residue that is left over after most of the mineral has been extracted may be stored in your body in places such as the joints and kidneys. Your body thinks you still have minerals available to draw on, so it excretes any additional minerals you swallow. But, because the stored minerals are attached to the carrier, they may not be bioavailable (absorbable) to the body, and you may become mineral deficient.

Electrolytes

Minerals in the brain create sparks called electrolytes. These charged particles are responsible for signals being delivered from one cell to the other. A salmon swimming upstream, when confronted with a waterfall, swims in circles at the base of the falling water. This helps the fish absorb the electrical charge created by the falling water and ultimately facilitates its miraculous leap up the waterfall. If electrolytes can do this for a fish, just think what they can do for your brain. On the other hand, if you are mineral deficient, your brain cannot create sparks and eventually short circuits. This can definitely hamper your ability to leap mental waterfalls or remember anything and everything.

Support Your Body
"GOOD" FAT—Surprise! It's great for your brain.

Low fat diets are designed to help your heart, but leaving out fats entirely or using the wrong type of fats can hurt your head. The brain is ten percent fat. "Good" fats support protection for the myelin sheath that surrounds the nerve fibers in the brain. If compromised, this covering can no longer provide protection against short circuits.

Choose "good" fats and avoid "bad" fats. Use reasonable amounts of select "good" fats to support your brain and body. Olive oil, butter, flax oil, borage, evening primrose and black currant oils provide the proper balance of omega-3 and omega-6 essential fatty acids. Essential fatty acids (EFA's) are necessary for the proper operation of cellular neurotransmitters. They are preferred to "bad" fats like margarine and most heated cooking oils, which may be hydrogenated or partially hydrogenated, and can clog arteries inside your body.

Choosing flax is one of the best ways to get essential fatty acids into your body. Flax oil can be used on salads as a dressing. However, it must be stored in a dark bottle in the refrigerator to avoid spoilage. Flax oil is available as a supplement, or an easy way to obtain your EFA's is to grind up flax seeds or buy them preground.

Flax contains an abundant balance of omega-3 and omega-6 essential fatty acids along with soluble and insoluble fiber and lignins. The nutrients in flax can give you quicker recovery from stress, improvement in behavioral disorders, mental clarity and calmness. Flax nutrients can foster learning ability and focus, enhance immune system function, and increase energy and stamina.

ENZYMES—Getting nutrients to the brain.

Enzymes are necessary to break down all nutrients we eat, including the "good" fats. Since most of us eat cooked foods, we are enzyme deficient. Many of the enzymes occurring naturally in raw food are killed during the heating process, and your body must then depend on the pancreas to produce what it needs.

Eventually this organ gets tired and produces less and less enzymes. This leads to undigested foods and the conditions associated with maldigestion, which include allergies, fatigue, and lethargy. Lipase is the enzyme needed to break down fats, therefore supplementation may be necessary to enhance absorption of the "good" fats that support your brain. When choosing an enzyme supplement it's best to pick one that says *plant enzymes* on the container. Plant enzymes work throughout the entire digestive tract, not just in the stomach.

BRAIN HAZARDS—The quick road to dementia.
Aspartame

Some ingredients added to the foods we eat are not part of Mother Nature's original recipe, and may be harmful to the body. The U.S Food and Drug Administration seems quick to approve food additives, and reluctant to take them out even after mountains of evidence shows that they can create illness and even death. One substance which has been studied at length is aspartame, the sugar substitute. Used to sweeten diet foods, this additive is now thought to create a craving for carbohydrates and may not help dieters at all.

At the World Environmental Conference in 1997, it was disclosed that when the temperature of aspartame exceeds 86°F, the wood alcohol in it converts to formaldehyde and then to formic acid (the poison found in the sting of fire ants), which in turn causes metabolic acidosis. The formaldehyde is stored in fat cells, particularly in the hips and thighs and is not easily removed. This methanol toxicity mimics multiple sclerosis. Therefore, many people diagnosed with MS may actually have Aspartame Disease. Aspartame has also been linked with a list of side effects which includes seizure, nausea, depression, migraine headaches, numbness and blindness.

Memory loss attributed to aspartame ingestion is due to the fact that aspartic acid and phenylalanine, which makes up aspartame, are neurotoxic when separated from the other amino acids found in protein. Thus it goes past the blood brain barrier and deteriorates the neurons of the brain. Dr. Russell Blaylock, neurosurgeon, says, "The ingredient stimulates the neurons of the brain to death, causing brain damage of varying degrees."[5] Dr. H.J. Roberts tells how aspartame poisoning is escalating Alzheimer's Disease. His diabetic patients presented memory loss, confusion and severe vision loss when they started on aspartame after it was first introduced.[6]

Soy

Another widely accepted food is soy. Rich in phytonutrients, soy is most beneficial when eaten in a fermented or sprouted form. The maturing of the soybean eliminates the trypsin (enzyme) inhibitor present in the whole bean. Raw soybeans, and foods made from them, may have difficulty being digested because of the enzyme inhibitor, and therefore their nutrients may not be available to the body.

Recently, certain soy products have been suspected in memory loss and brain damage in men and unborn children. Made from *unsprouted* soy, these soy products have difficulty being digested through normal enzymatic processes. The body, in an effort to rid itself of this food, uses minerals as carriers for the elimination process. If enough unfermented soy is eaten, this process reduces mineral levels in the body. We speculate that this could cause memory loss, because as stated previously, minerals are essential for proper brain function.

Table Sugar

Common table sugar can also have an adverse effect on our brains. According to Sabina Wise in her book, *The Sugar Addict's Diet*, "we can get the sugar dumbs." Sabrina goes on to say, "Problems with cognitive function are a direct result of insufficient fuels to the nervous system. Detecting a high blood sugar

[5]Blalock, R.L., M.D., Excitotoxins, *The Taste That Kills*, Health Press, 1997.
[6]Roberts, Dr. H.J., *Defense Against Alzheimer's Disease*, Sunshine Sentinel Press, 1995.

level alerts the pancreas to secrete insulin to lower the blood sugar and shortly the adrenal glands send cortisol into the blood to raise the blood sugar again.

Cortisol can actually cause damage to the hippocampus—our memory center. In maintaining the blood sugar balance, which has been upset by an infusion of sugar, the brain takes a direct hit. Low blood sugar symptoms can appear within twenty minutes of eating sugar and result in mental and emotional disturbances as well as short-term memory problems.

Aluminum

Aluminum is present in many foods we ingest, such as baking powder and in drinking water—another good reason for a water filter. Toxicity, from cooking with aluminum pots and pans, can induce symptoms such as a lack of coordination. Aluminum has been suspected in contributing to diseases such as Alzheimer's. Aluminum in the body results in an *electrolyte imbalance* and disrupts vital body functions, which can lead to disease conditions. If you suspect an overabundance of aluminum in your body, you may chelate (remove through a carrier) this metal and excrete it by taking large amounts of trace minerals and Vitamin C. As with any such protocol, ask the advice of a health practitioner prior to self-treatment.

Electromagnetic Devices

Activities such as playing computer games may be detrimental to the brain because of fields created by electromagnetic energy. These fields work at a different frequency than the human body, which tries to convert them to a harmonious cycle. The effort expended in this process not only compromises the immune system, but adds stress to the brain, reducing its effectiveness. Computers (with cathode ray tube monitors), video games, electric blankets, cell phones and televisions all provide electromagnetic frequencies that can negatively affect the user.

It is wise to investigate the many protective devices that are sold, such as elemental diodes and cathode ray tube shields. For maximum protection, make sure the user sits three feet away from the television or computer (keyboard with long cord), use electric blankets only to prewarm the bed and minimize usage of cellular phones, which have been implicated in ear and jawbone cancer.

According to panelists at the Cell Tower Forum presented by the Berkshire-Litchfield Environmental Council in Connecticut, cell phone frequencies have been shown, in laboratory studies to cause intermittent release of calcium from brain tissue. This may result in difficulties with memory, motor coordination and neurotransmitter function.

EXERCISE
Midline crossing movements.

Exercises that cross a line from head to toe separating the left and right sides of your body stimulate the neurons in the brain. Neural development begins when we are babies. The first movements that cross the midline, like sucking, rolling over and crawling, encourage brain development. Sitting in a car or at a computer for hours does not.

Activities that integrate physical and mental functions can be beneficial if they use midline crossing movements such as playing ping-pong, golf, badminton or tennis; doing Nia techniques, Tai Chi, Yoga or Kung Fu. Beneficial activities also include playing chess, doing puzzles, sweeping floors or swinging your arms across your midline while walking. Activities that do not further neural development are those that require sitting still for long periods of time like driving, computer work, or watching TV. Physical movements stimulate the brain, therefore the more we move, the smarter we become and have less chances for *senior moments* to appear.

Stress inhibits neural function, therefore any technique that calms you can have a beneficial effect on memory. When normal brain function is impaired through inactivity, learning disabilities and communication difficulties may appear.

In order to stay sharp, we must coordinate:
   A. the left cerebral hemisphere of the brain with the right, which affects our reading ability and communication;
   B. the higher and lower parts of the brain essential for feeling and the expression of emotions;
   C. focusing the back and front lobes of the brain, which keeps brain function in context and prevents attention and comprehension disorders.

Specific movements have been defined that stimulate or relax our neural pathways in the brain. Educational Kinesiology was developed in the early 1980s by Dr. Paul E. Dennison, and has grown into a system of exercises for the brain called *Brain Gym.* These twenty-three movements are based on over twenty-five years of research and are endorsed by the National Learning Foundation. *Brain Gym* movements and exercises integrate the brain's various dimensions allowing information to flow easily from sense into memory and then out again. An example of one exercise is to visualize the letter X.

Brain Gym activates the brain for whole body coordination and increases concentration. If you are having learning or recall difficulties, we suggest you explore this exercise program for the brain. The Educational Kinesiology Foundation can be contacted at 800.356.2109 or on-line at *www.braingym.org.*

"Hi, S-naps again!
That's the nitty-gritty—now for
some suggestions on supplements
and substances that can act as
brain boosters."

Supplements

Supplements that help
Amino Acids
Betaine
Chiropractic
CoQ10
DHA
Flower remedies

Herbal Brain Boosters
Ginkgo biloba
Gotu Kola
Rosemary
Rhodiola rosea
Hormone balancing
Lecithin
Phosphidityl serine
Phosphiditylcholine
Minerals
Magnesium
Sulfur
Zinc
Vitamins
E
B_1
B_{12}
Velvet antler

In addition to the basic brain support protocol outlined in Chapter Three, we list various supplements that may help individual cases. Increasing levels of mineralized water, enzymes and essential fatty acids will give everyone's brain the tools for improved operation. The following suggestions are to be considered additional remedies for specific conditions. They should be chosen only after receiving a proper diagnosis of your condition from a health practitioner.

Amino Acids

Amino acids are necessary to keep your brain's neurotransmitters firing properly. Part of an aging brain's failing memory problem is recalling information. Supporting your brain with DL-phenylalanine and L-Glutamine, two key amino acids, will provide the ammunition your body needs to repair or rebuild failing neural signals.

Phenylalanine is an essential amino acid that helps you feel happy and motivated. Glutamine is a conditionally essential amino acid that can keep you calm, focused and in control. In order to function properly, your body must have the essential amino acid, phenylalanine. *(Please note that the natural food supplement DL-phenylalanine should not be confused with the chemically altered form of phenylalanine which is in the artificial sweetener, aspartame.)*

Stress, insufficient diet, alcohol and drug abuse can deplete your body of amino acids. In addition to failing memory, lack of neurotransmitter support can cause depression, fatigue, anxiety and feelings of hopelessness that have normally been associated with *just getting old.* Since your body cannot convert amino acids from other nutrients, it must depend on outside sources and specific supplements to acquire sufficient amounts.

These key amino acids are found in cold water, white fish. Amino acids from meat, eggs and dairy sources cannot readily be utilized by your brain because they do not contain the cofactors (helper substances), which help them cross the blood brain barrier. It is necessary to take supplements which contain these cofactors. One such supplement is Rhodiola rosea herbal extract. Tests have shown the quality of a task performed by the brain is dependent on fatigue levels. When Rhodiola was administered, it effectively increased a person's resistance to fatigue, enhanced back muscle strength, hand-strength endurance and improved coordination.

A nonessential amino acid that your body can produce if given the proper tools is L-carnitine. These tools are Vitamin B_1, B_6, C, iron, lysine and methionine. L-carnitine is found mainly in the brain, heart and skeletal muscles. It plays a vital role in delivering fatty acids to the mitochondria, which supplies power for the cells, allowing them to better utilize oxygen. L-carnitine may be helpful in treating Alzheimer's disease patients by slowing, preventing or reversing the disease. A common sign of L-carnitine deficiency is mental confusion and muscle weakness. Found mostly in dairy products, meats, fermented soy and grains fortified with lysine, such as cornmeal, it is also available in supplement form. (*Note: Look for L-carnitine as it is better absorbed and has no side effects as compared to D-carnitine.*)

E "Supplements"
Betaine (TMG)

Found in animals and plants, mostly in spinach, beets and broccoli, Betaine is also known as trimethylglycine (TMG). It is a substance that turns the potentially dangerous amino acid homocysteine into beneficial methionine. Other substances that can do this are SAMe, Vitamin B_{15}, B_3, B_6 and folic acid. As we age, our homocysteine levels increase resulting in increased chances of developing arthritis, depression, Alzheimer's and certain cancers. Betaine and omega-3 essential fatty acids, along with the others mentioned above, help reduce homocysteine levels.

Chiropractic

Surprising as it may sound, chiropractic treatment may help overcome *senior moments*. During a lifetime we all experience falls, jarring bumps in cars and planes, twisting strains, sitting doing tasks for hours or even stressful emotional outbreaks. These episodes can cause your back or neck to get *a crook* in it. If not corrected, misalignment can develop into a chronic condition that we accept and just learn to live with. Dr. Ogi Ressel, says, "Decreased nerve and blood supply to the brain leads to an inability of the body to function properly manifesting as degenerative conditions such as Alzheimer's, senility, memory loss, irritability, and depression. All of these conditions are a result of interference in the brain's ability to communicate with the rest of the body."[7]

When the vertebrae of the neck becomes misaligned (subluxation), it decreases the size of the holes between the vertebrae where the nerves lie. This pinching type action causes pressure on the nerves and on the blood vessels decreasing blood to the

[7]Ressel, Dr. Ogi., Kids First, *Health with No Interference*, New Century Publishing 2000, 2001.

brain. According to Dr. Ogi Ressel, D.C., and author of *Kids First*, "a vertebral subluxation is an irritant to the nervous system. It is similar to having a pebble placed in your shoe that you can't get rid of."[8] Chiropractic care is directed at correcting these subluxations. It helps the nervous system function normally, by increasing blood flow resulting in reduced brain trauma.

CoQ10

Co-enzyme Q10 is one of the most potent antioxidants that protects the body from free-radical damage. It plays a critical role in energy production at the cellular level and is instrumental in oxygen delivery to the cells. Deficiencies can be dietary, with sources coming from fish and meat, but may also be caused by a synthesis malfunction in the body. Studies show that mitochondrial function appears to be impaired in Alzheimer's patients. Due to CoQ10's beneficial effects on this mitochondrial functioning, it has prevented the progression of the disease for one to two years. CoQ10 in supplement form is absorbed better when taken with "good" fat.

DHA

Ducosahexaenoic acid (DHA) is an essential fatty acid which is necessary for neurological development in infants, and its need may extend into adulthood, especially during times of stress. DHA is effective in protecting against peroxisomal disorders which damage the myelin sheath, the protective covering surrounding nerves. Studies have confirmed that there is a definite link between Alzheimer's and a deficiency of DHA.

Found in cold water fish such as mackerel, salmon, herring, sardines, black cod, anchovies, albacore tuna, and cod liver oil, it can also be obtained in supplement form. Since fish oil is damaged by oxygen, when choosing a supplement, select brands that include Vitamin E, which protects the oil from the free-radical and oxidation damage.

Flower remedies

Many emotional problems associated with memory failure can

---

[8]Ressel, Dr. Ogi., KIDS FIRST, *Health with No Interference*, New Century Publishing 2000, 2001.

be treated with flower remedies. Flower remedies can be effective in cases where there are feelings of discouragement, failure, insecurity, lethargy and frustration.

People with a lack of concentration may be helped by clematis. Those who are discouraged can be helped by gentian. Motivation may be bolstered through wild rose. These remedies are commonly administered through tinctures placed under the tongue and work within minutes.

Herbal Brain Boosters

THE INFORMATION IN THIS SECTION WAS WRITTEN BY LAUREL DEWEY, AUTHOR OF THE HUMOROUS HERBALIST AND PLANT POWER.[9]

While the herbs listed below have been shown over centuries to improve brain function—either by increasing circulatory action to the head or via preserving the vital tissues and nerve centers in the brain—it is important to understand that these plant medicines *may not combine safely* with some prescription drugs. Some herbs may increase the action of the drug or shorten the drug's transit time in your bloodstream. Furthermore, if you choose *standardized*, also known as *guaranteed potency*, herbal preparations, the effect on the body in tandem with prescription drugs may be magnified. Be certain to check with your physician or holistic healthcare provider before taking any of these herbs along with your medication.

Ginkgo biloba

Known as the longevity herb, ginkgo regenerates the body by stimulating blood flow, particularly to the brain and the legs. With this *shot of circulation*, there is a burst of oxygen which may account for a renewed ability to think more clearly and move more easily. For about sixty percent of the people who partake of ginkgo, there is a marked improvement in circulation, nervous system activity and the ability to concentrate.

A study in the *Journal of the American Medical Association* concluded that Ginkgo biloba extract alleviated the symptoms associated with a range of cognitive disorders, and was beneficial in the treatment of dementia. It concluded that this herb was safe and appears capable of stabilizing and improving the cognitive

[9]Dewey, Laurel, *The Humorous Herbalist*, East Canaan, CT, Safe Goods 1997; Dewey, Laurel, *Plant Power*, East Canaan, CT, New Century Publishing 2000.

performance and the social functioning of demented patients for six months to one year.[10]

In a study done in the 1980s, 112 geriatric patients ranging in age from 55 to 94 were given 40 mgs of *standardized* ginkgo extract three times per day. After one year, all of the people showed minor to massive improvement when it came to memory, headaches, depression and concentration. The scientists wanted to see what would happen if they gave the same dose to eight young, healthy women, and then gave them a memory test. All tested higher after ingesting ginkgo extract.

One interesting experiment showed that a man who took 40 mgs of *standardized* ginkgo, up to one hour before studying, was able to retain more information and stay focused, even when studying far into the night. Another study showed that continuous doses of ginkgo on a daily basis appeared to halt deterioration of people who were just beginning to have memory lapses. Four double-blind studies have shown that ginkgo is helpful for people in the early stages of Alzheimer's and other forms of Dementia including Multi-infarct Dementia.

In Europe, ginkgo is being given to Alzheimer's patients and findings show that it is helping to create alertness as well as slow down the effects of the disease. Ginkgo can be taken in liquid extract or capsule form.

A note of caution: Since ginkgo has the ability to reduce blood clotting, if you have a clotting disorder, check with your health practitioner before taking the herb. Beware of overdosing in hopes of becoming **younger by Thursday,** *as you may experience nausea, diarrhea and vomiting.*

Gotu Kola

Research literature from India calls gotu kola, *food for the brain,* because it stimulates the brain as it encourages and builds what the East Indian calls *Prana*—The Life Force. Researchers have been able to break down the active compounds in gotu kola, but many admit they still aren't sure how it accomplishes everything it does. Evidence shows that, like ginkgo biloba, it enhances the circulatory system. In addition, gotu kola has been shown to combat fatigue,

[10]Journal of the American Medical Association, October 22, 1997.

enhance learning and comprehension, and improve the ability to focus. It has slowed the progress and improved the quality of life in Alzheimer's patients, helped control some of the jittery symptoms of Parkinson's disease, alleviated some forms of depression and acted as both a preventive and treatment for those who suffer nervous breakdowns. Gotu kola is available in liquid or capsule form and can be taken indefinitely. To jump start the mental effect of gotu kola, it helps to combine it in equal parts with ginkgo biloba.

Beware of the side effects of high doses, which may include throbbing headaches, feeling out of one's body, and the increased need to scratch one's skin. If you suffer from hyperthyroidism (overactive thyroid), there is information that claims the use of gotu kola aggravates the condition. On the other hand, if you have an underactive thyroid, it may help, as long as you do not use it if you are taking glandular medication. Do not confuse gotu kola with the caffeine-rich kola nut herb. They are not the same.

Rosemary

Centuries ago, people discovered that by wrapping meat in layers of crushed rosemary leaves, it stayed fresher longer. This reputation for preservation had many people leaping to the conclusion that rosemary could also preserve the memory. They may not have been that far off.

Rosemary has been shown to contain approximately twenty-four known antioxidants, the compounds that slow the aging process at the cellular level. This is why rosemary works so well as a natural meat preservative. Oxidative damage in the body can lead to tissue disintegration and diseases such as Alzheimer's. Studies show that several of the antioxidant compounds in rosemary have proven equal in strength to synthetic antioxidants such as BHA and BHT. Rosemary is easily ingested as a tea or tincture, but excessive internal doses of fresh or dried rosemary can cause stomach cramps and even slight poisoning. Beware that rosemary tea can bring on menstruation. For this reason, *pregnant women should not use rosemary in tea or liquid form.* A sprig or two to season your food is fine, as long as the meat isn't packed in the herb.

Rhodiola rosea

Exactly how extracts of the Rhodiola rosea plant influences learning and memory is still a topic of debate. According to contemporary notions, the process of memory formation is supported by the interactions between various neurotransmitters in the brain.

The role of serotonin activated neurons transmission during the learning process, and the formation of memory, is well known. But other neurotransmitters in the brain are also important. The role of neurotransmitter systems may be different depending on the nature of the learning process. As an example, some animals, whose serotonin levels have been reduced, show no significant changes in the learning process, while other animal experiments show improved status.

A few Russian researchers have found that a moderate decrease of the neurotransmitter, norepinephrine (noradrenaline), improves the learning and memory processes. Subsequent studies have shown that salidroside, an extract of Rhodiola, moderately lowers the amount of norepinephrine and dopamine in the brain. Rhodiola can effectively modulate levels of norepinephrine, which plays a critical role in the stress response. The latter theory may explain how this herb influences intellectual capacity.

To test the duration of Rhodiola's effect, investigators observed two treatment groups one, two, three, four, six, eight and twenty-four hours after taking ten drops of the preparation. After one hour, those not taking Rhodiola rosea experienced a thirteen percent increase in the number of errors made. By the fourth hour the number of errors increased by thirty-seven percent, the sixth hour eighty-eight percent, and by the eighth hour, a whopping 180 percent increase was observed. In the group taking Rhodiola, a fifty-six percent decrease in the number of errors was observed, and this effect lasted four hours. After that, the percentage of errors made increased, but to a lesser extent than in the group not taking Rhodiola rosea.

Investigators concluded the preparation of Rhodiola improved intellectual work capacity after a one-time dose, being reflected primarily in the quality of work performed. The stimulating effect of Rhodiola is also clearly manifested in the performance of mental work.[11]

[11]This section reprinted from: *Stress and Weight Management Using Rhodiola Rosea and Rhododendron Caucasicum* by Dr. Zakir Ramazanov and Dr. Maria del Mar Bernal Suarez, Safe Goods, 1999.

Hormone balancing

The body has created a myriad of hormones that affect body function, mood and our health. Both men and women produce estrogen and progesterone and any time nature's balance of these hormones is upset, both sexes can develop problems.

Excess estrogen is associated with heart problems, stroke and hypoxia, the lack of oxygen. An overabundance of estrogen promotes thyroid deficiencies because it inhibits thyroid secretion. This results in many symptoms, but those that target brain function are headaches, insomnia, fatigue, depression, constipation and cancer.

You may be getting excess estrogen through your food and your environment. Many chemicals like chlorine, pesticides and PCBs, which are petroleum by-products, are thought to mimic estrogen in the body, creating mixed messages. The brain compensates for this excess estrogen and creates symptoms that are identical to those for actual hormonal imbalances.

Menopausal women who embark on hormone replacement therapy should check with a healthcare professional and monitor their estrogen levels carefully, especially if they are prone to exposure of environmental *estrogenic* substances. Because progesterone balances estrogen, these women should always take supplemental (transdermal) natural progesterone to keep estrogen levels in check. Progesterone is best taken through the skin as a cream application, since it is very poorly absorbed orally. Natural progesterone is far more harmonious with the body than synthetic prescription brands, and will rarely cause any side effects. Hormone balancing with natural progesterone may exhibit physical benefits such as improved memory, reduced foggy thinking, minimized headaches, eliminated depression and lowered mood swings.

Many herbs can also assist in balancing the hormones. Dong Quai is a bittersweet herb that is widely used in the Orient as a tonic for the female reproductive system. Dong Quai has a regulating and normalizing effect on hormone production. Maca, Licorice, Chaste Tree Berry and Black Cohosh are other herbs that may be considered support for hormone functions.

Lecithin

Lecithin is produced by our livers and is essential to brain function. It is made up of Choline, Linoleic acid and Inositol, which are successful in crossing the blood-brain barrier, a necessity to nourish brain cells.

In his book, *The Memory Solution,* Dr. Julian Whitaker, M.D., explains that lecithin is the major source of the neurotransmitter, acetylcholine, which determines human behavior and is the most important substance in nerve transmission. It is particularly needed by the brain for repair and maintenance. As we age, acetylcholine levels decline, leading to a reduction in both short and long-term memory.[12]

As an essential fatty acid it also helps lower blood pressure and regulate cholesterol levels. Deficiencies can hamper the proper operation of the brain. In *Prescriptions for Nutritional Healing,* James Balch, M.D., tells us that the protective sheaths surrounding the brain are composed of lecithin, as are the muscles and nerves. Therefore, maintaining adequate levels of lecithin can help to reduce the mental symptoms associated with aging. Extracted from egg yolks and soybeans, lecithin is easy to come by as a supplement.[13]

LECITHIN-DERIVED SUPPLEMENTS:
Phosphatidyl Serine (PS)

The brain's remarkable ability to perceive and perform, remember and learn, is severely challenged by today's social and physical environment. These factors accelerate the decline in nerve cell activity that normally occurs with age.

Phosphatidyl Serine (PS) is a phospholipid which forms an essential part in every human cell, but it is particularly concentrated in the membranes of nerve cells. Unlike other cells in the body, nerve cells do not reproduce. Instead, they repair and rebuild themselves, using proteins called Nerve Growth Factor (NGF). PS enhances the synthesis and reception of NGF and supports brain functions that tend to diminish with age.

---

[12] Whitaker, Dr. Julian M., *The Memory Solution: Dr. Julian Whitaker's 10-Step Program to Optimize Your Memory and Brain Function,* with Peggy Dance, Garden City Park, NY, Avery Publishing Group, 1999.

[13] Balch, James R., M.D., Phyllis A. Balch, PRESCRIPTIONS FOR NUTRITIONAL HEALING: An A-Z Guide to Supplements, Garden City Park, NY, Avery Publishing Group, 1998.

PS, related to lecithin, also may be related to the body's response to stress, as taking a PS supplement appears to produce fewer stress hormones in response to exercise-induced stress. PS may have the potential to minimize a common problem in today's world— stress induced memory lapse. PS improves mental function. Studies with higher does per day showed people more able to remember names and recall misplaced objects.[14]

Phosphatidylcholine

In order for information to be processed in the brain, we must depend on neurons to communicate with each other through a chemical process. When a neuron sends a signal to another neuron, a transmitter chemical is released. These neurotransmitting brain chemicals depend not only on water but on fat chemicals and associated nutrients. Acetylcholine is one of the neurotransmitters that brain cells use to communicate with each other. Acetylcholine controls the rate of the stimulus entering the brain, it also controls motor activity and memory, and is essential in maintaining brain cell structure.

Aging causes a decline in the levels of neurotransmitters such as acetylcholine, because of the brain's diminishing ability to make these chemicals. Aging also causes an increase of enzymes that destroy acetylcholine. This lack of acetylcholine may be one cause of memory problems and *senior moments.*[14]

Older brains normally show shrinkage and exhibit the neurofibrillary tangles associated with senility, resulting in memory loss. It has been suggested that by taking extra choline throughout life, you may slow the aging process of the brain.[15] Phosphatidylcholine, an active ingredient in soy lecithin, similar to PS, can help restore adequate levels of acetylcholine.

Choline exists in abundant levels in newborn babies where it is necessary for the manufacture of myelin, the material that insulates and protects the nervous system. Studies have provided evidence that choline may improve other brain functions that don't use acetylcholine as a neurotransmitter, such as those that control body coordination.

[14]Schmidt, R., Hayn, M., Reinhart, B., et al, PLASMA ANTIOXIDANT AND COGNITIVE PERFORMANCE IN MIDDLE-AGED AND OLDER ADULTS: *Results of the Austrian Stroke Prevention Study*; Jamaeriat Soc., 1998; 46: 1407-10.

[15]UNIQUE NATURAL COMBINATIONS OF GINKGO AND PHOSPHATIDYLCHOLINE, *Life Extension Magazine*, May 1988, www.lef.org/magazine.

Every cell membrane in the body requires phosphatidylcholine (PC). Nerve and brain cells need large quantities of PC for repair and maintenance. It also is instrumental in the metabolism of fats, regulating blood cholesterol, and specific to the brain, nourishes the fat-like sheaths of the brain's nerve fibers. PC is a primary source of the neurotransmitter acetylcholine, which is used by the brain in areas that control long-term planning, concentration and focus.

Foods contain only trace amounts of free choline. It is mostly found in lecithin, which can help increase choline levels. When supplementing with choline or lecithin PC, you can increase the amount of acetylcholine available for memory and our thought process. DMAE (2-dimethylaminoethanol) may also increase levels of the brain neurotransmitter acetylcholine. The acetyl group part of acetyl-L-carnitine also contributes to the production of acetylcholine. Several clinical trials suggested that acetyl-L-carnitine delays the progression of Alzheimer's, improves memory and enhances the patient's performance.[16]

MINERALS
THE FOLLOWING INDIVIDUAL MINERALS ARE SUPPLEMENTAL TO THE BASIC TRACE MINERALS REFERRED TO IN CHAPTER THREE.

Magnesium
A contributing factor to memory loss is the calcification of the brain tissue leading to nerve cell death. In part, this is caused by an upset in the calcium-magnesium balance in your body. With all the hype on taking calcium for strong bones, we have overlooked the fact that our body chemistry may be upset if not balanced with magnesium. When too much calcium is deposited in an area of the body, it is called calcification. Calcification of brain tissue can affect neural functioning. Magnesium is also the antistress mineral and is essential for proper nerve function.

Symptoms of deficiency can be confusion, disorientation, nervousness and anger. Contributors to a deficiency are alcohol, coffee, chronic stress, sugar, milk containing synthetic Vitamin D,

[16]Pettegrew, J.W., Klunk, W.E., Panchalingam, K. et al, *Clinical and neurochemical effects of acetyl-L-carnitine treatment of neural decline in the elderly*, Drugs Exp Clin Res, 1994, 20:169-76.

and drugs such as oral contraceptives, tetracyclines, antibiotics and diuretics. Natural sources of magnesium are almonds, honey, green vegetables, kelp, seafood, spinach, soy and wheat bran. When selecting a magnesium supplement, choose an ionic form as this small size will maximize bioavailability to the cells and reduce chances of toxicity.

Sulfur

Nutritional sulfur is required by many functions of the body. Specifically necessary for the brain, sulfur helps to repair the myelin sheath that protects our nerves. Natural sources of sulfur are bran, cheese, clams, eggs, fish, garlic, nuts, onion and wheat germ. Supplemental forms of sulfur are best obtained in an ionic form to maximize absorption.

Zinc

Zinc has been known to help optimize brain function and promote mental alertness. An essential mineral, zinc acts as an antioxidant and has been helpful in treating Alzheimer's disease. Natural sources of zinc are nutritional yeast, liver, mushrooms, seafood, soy, spinach, sunflower seeds and whole grains. If you decide to take a zinc supplement, purchase it in the smallest molecular form (ionic), as this assures delivery into the cells where it can do its work. Smaller molecules also protect against toxicity, as the body can easily eliminate excessive quantities. Deficiencies in zinc may occur from alcohol, high calcium intake and lack of phosphorus along with drugs such as diuretics.

VITAMINS
Vitamin E

This vitamin, a high antioxidant, has been shown to slow the progression of Alzheimer's. In a study of 341 people with Alzheimer's, a 2000 IU dose of Vitamin E per day extended the period of time they were able to care for themselves, during the progression of the disease. [17]

---

[17]Sano M., Ernesto, C. Thomas, R. A., et al, *A Controlled Trial of Seleginine Alpha-Tocopherol or both as Treatment for Alzheimer's Disease*, N.E. Jnl. of Med., 1997; 336:1216-22.

Higher Vitamin E levels are known to correspond with better brain function in middleaged adults. Vitamin E is found naturally in dark green vegetables, eggs, wheat germ, peanuts and tomatoes. Deficiencies can be caused by low utilization precipitated by birth control pills, chlorine in water, rancid fats and low zinc levels.

Vitamin B$_1$ (Thiamine)

This B vitamin is involved in the process of nerve transmissions within sections of the brain called cholinergic neurons that deteriorate in Alzheimer's patients. Decreased activity of Vitamin B$_1$ dependent enzymes in these patients is the suspected reason. It is thought that by supplementing with B$_1$, the progression of Alzheimer's may be slowed.

Deficiencies can be caused by substances that prevent the maximum utilization of this vitamin by the body. These include alcohol, antacids, baking soda, caffeine, raw fish, excessive sugar, stress and heat from cooking. Some medications such as Tagamet, diuretics, tetracyclines and cough syrups containing caffeine may also contribute to deficiencies. Vitamin B$_1$ is found in nutritional yeast, peanuts, sunflower seeds, brown rice, fish, meat, whole grains and wheat germ.

Vitamin B$_{12}$

B$_{12}$ and folic acid (folacin B complex) have also been shown to be deficient in people with Alzheimer's. Vitamin B$_{12}$ supports the nervous system and plays a key part in mental functioning. B$_{12}$ deficiencies can be caused by certain drugs such as birth control pills, topical steroids and sulfonamides, and can stem from dietary deficiencies. B$_{12}$ is most commonly found in nutritional yeast, milk, eggs, tuna, liver and cottage cheese. Symptoms of deficiency may be anxiety, depression, difficulties in walking and speaking, and general weakness.

Folic acid deficiencies may be caused by stress and the use of alcohol, coffee and tobacco along with medications such as barbiturates, oral contraceptives, and sulfonamides and topical steroids. Folic Acid is found in nutritional yeast, dates, spinach, tuna fish, citrus fruits, beets, green leafy vegetables, milk and salmon.

Velvet Antler

Neurotransmitters in the brain such as dopamine, serotonin and norepinephrine can be broken down because of an enzyme function, MAO (monoamine oxidase). Velvet antler, as a supplement, can significantly inhibit these MAO enzymes, and thus protect the brain from neurotransmitter damage.

Velvet Antler is a humanely harvested "hormonizing" remedy from elk or deer antlers. Used clinically in Russian since the 1930s, this complex substance has recently been made available in the rest of the world. It is an effective anti-inflammatory, immune stimulant and growth stimulator, has been used to increase athletic strength and endurance and is considered an aphrodisiac.

*"That's it—in words and pictures. Now get out there and take charge of **your** neural circuitry!"*

Meiser

Frances Meiser is an educator, author and pioneer bringing new information on brain function and its' neuroplasticity to the educational arena and an aging population.

At age fifty she was labeled with Attention Deficit Hyperactivity Disorder. That ordeal, and her personal experiences with panic attacks, drove her to seek help from The HANDLE Institute.® With the aid of their training, she moved beyond these dysfunctions to discover, "a brightness I never knew I had."

Intensive study led her to a layman's understanding of how the brain develops and continues to develop and change throughout life. Her integrated, holistic, practical approach to daily brain maintenance for all ages is being cheered by parents, educators and the business community.

She is the author of *The Brain Train*, an easy-to-read book for children on brain care, and Executive Director of The Brain Train Center, a nonprofit organization that teaches "healthy habits make healthy brains." Her presentations at a variety of conferences have helped people unlock *their* hidden potential, create new brain pathways and experience less stress and more joy in their lives.

Ms. Meiser holds a Bachelor's Degree in Elementary Education and Early Child Development and is completing a Master's Degree in Language and Literacy in Austin, Texas.

Anderson

Nina Anderson is an International Sports Science Association Certified Specialist in Performance Nutrition. She has authored fourteen books on natural health for people and animals, including the best-selling *ADD, The Natural Approach.*

She has spent the last twenty years in the natural health arena. A frequent guest on radio and television shows She frequently lectures on the subject of Attention Deficit

Biographies

Disorder and anti-aging. Nina is Vice-President of Safe Goods/New Century Publishing 2000 and President of the nonprofit organization, The Scientific Alliance for Education.

Bossard

Yvonne Cecile Bossard is an award-winning designer and Creative Director of ART ALaCarte Austin, a traditional/digital illustration and graphic design firm. She is an instructor in the Digital Publishing and Graphics Technology Department at Austin Community College in Austin, Texas.

She received a Silver *Award of Excellence*, Texas Graphic Excellence Award for the Central Texas Recycling Associations 1999 Annual Report and a Bronze *Award of Merit*, Texas Graphic Excellence Award for the Women's Chamber of Commerce of Texas MAPCON 199: Women of the Century mailer.

Yvonne has more than twenty years of experience in fine art, illustration and graphic design and holds a Bachelor's Degree in Fine Art and Journalism. She is a member of the Graphic Artists Guild and the Women's Chamber of Commerce of Texas.

© 2001 The Brain Train Center

Aarisse, P.O. Box 210, Oakland, NJ 07436
800.675.9329, **www. aarisse.com**
Natural progesterone, hormone testing kits.

Alpha-Lyte, P.O. Box 531, Jenison, MI 49429-0531
888-NUTRITION, 888.688.7484
Bottled water with trace mineral electrolytes.

Alternate Health, P.O. Box 5351,
Lake Montezuma, AZ 86342
800.233.0810, **www.alternatehealth.net**
Flower remedies for memory, concentration and focus.

Alternatives Direct, P.O. Box 25, Windham,
NH 03087-0025, 800.258.5014
Antioxidant and memory enhancing supplements.

Ameriden, P.O. Box 1870, Fallbrook, CA 92088
888.405.3336, **www.2ameriden.com**
*Supplements that contain high antioxidants, anti-aging
properties, memory enhancers, neurotransmitter support
fat blockers and fat releasers.*

ATN Products, 561 Shunpike Rd., Sheffield, MA 01257,
888.217.7233
*Highly absorbable ionic efforescent minerals for antiaging,
brain and immune support.*

Fountain of Youth, P.O. Box 608, Millersport, OH
43046, 800.939.4296
*Supplements for anti-aging, anxiety reduction and growth
hormone enhancing.*

The HANDLE Institute®, 1530 Eastlake Ave. E.,
Suite 100, Seattle, WA 98102, 206.860.2665,
fax: 206.860.3505, e-mail: support@handle.org,
www.handle.org
*Nonprofit training and research organization for ADD, LD,
Tourette's syndrome, brain injury, stroke, Cerebral Palsy,
autism, memory problems, language delays.*

Heintzman Farms, RR2, P.O. Box 265,
Onaka, SD 57466
800.333.5813, **www.heintzmanfarms.com**
Flaxseed fresh from the farm and ready to grind.
(Send a self-addressed, stamped envelope for a sample.)

Natural Ovens Bakery of Manitowoc, Wisconsin,
4300 Country Trunk CR., P.O. Box 730,
Manitowoc, WI 54221-0730
800.558.3535, **www.naturalovens.com**
Fortified flaxseed as ingredient in bread, bagels, rolls,
cereals, mixes and muffins.

Nature's Path, P.O. Box 7862, Venice, FL 34287-7862
800.326-5772, **www.naturespathinc.com**
Trace minerals and full supplement line for anti-aging,
immune support, including lecithin for brain health.

New Wave Enviro, P.O. Box 4146, Englewood, CO 80155,
800.592.8371
Water filtration products for shower, refrigerators, ten-stage
drinking water filtration with KDF.

Omega-Life Inc., P.O. Box 208, Brookfield,
WI 53009-0298, 1.262.786.2070, 1.800.EAT-FLAX
1.800.328.3529, **www.fortifiedflax.com**
Fortified flaxmeal, drink mix for brain support,
flax nutrition bars.

Prozyme, 6444 N. Ridgeway Ave., Lincolnwood, IL 60712,
800.522.5537
Bioavailable digestive plant enzymes.

Wakunaga of America, 23501 Madero, Mission Viejo,
CA 92691, 800.825.7888
Aged garlic extract, greens and acidophilus for immune
support. Neurologic supplement for brain health.

Anderson, Nina; Peiper, Dr. N. Howard; *A.D.D., The Natural Approach,* Safe Goods Publishing, East Canaan, CT, 1996.

Austin American Statesman, October 1998. Adapted from *All–Mozart Music Diet Turns Lab Rats Into Maze Busters,* Joseph B. Verrengia, A.P., October 4, 1998.

Balch, James F., M.D., Phyllis A. Balch, *Prescriptions for Nutritional Healing: An A–Z Guide to Supplements,* Garden City Park, NY, Avery Publishing Group, 1998.

Barnett, Anthony, *Soya alert over cancer and brain damage link,* Guardian Newspapers Ltd. (www.observer.co.uk), August 2000.

Batmanghelidj, F.; *Your Body's Many Cries for Water.,* Global Health Solutions, Falls Church, VA, 1997.

Bell, Rachel, Peiper, H., *The A.D.D and A.D.H.D DIET!,* East Canaan, CT, Safe Goods, 1997.

Blalock, R.L., M.D., *Excitotoxins, The Taste That Kills,* Health Press, 1997.

Bluestone, Judith, *NOT YOUR ORDINARY WORKOUT: The HANDLE Institute® Creates Unusual Exercises to Treat Attention Deficit Disorder, Autism.,* Puget Sound Business Journal (David Volk), 23-29, May 1997.

Dennison, Dr. Paul E., *Switching On: A Guide to Edu-Kinesthetics,* The Educational Kinesiology Foundation Glendale, CA, 1981.

Dewey, Laurel, *The Humorous Herbalist,* East Canaan, CT, Safe Goods Publishing and *Plant Power,* East Canaan, CT, New Century Publishing 2000.

Bibliography

Hannaford, Carla, Ph.D, SMART MOVES–*Why Learning Is Not All In Your Head,* Great Ocean Publishers, Arlington, VA, 1995.

Health After 50, John's Hopkins Medical Letters, July, 1996.

Journal of the American Medical Association, October 22, 1997.

Le Bars, P.L., Katz, M.M., Brennan, N., et al, *A placebo controlled double-blind randomized trial of an extract of Ginkgo biloba for dementia,* North Am EGB Study Group, JAMA, 1997, 278:327-32.

Life Extension: UNIQUE NATURAL COMBINATIONS OF GINKGO AND PHOSPHATIDYLCHOLINE, *Life Extension Magazine,* May 1988, www.lef.org/magazine.

Mackintosh, Nicolas, Treays, Rebecca, *Understanding Your Brain,* Usborne Science for Beginners, EDC Publishing, Tulsa, OK, 1996.

McCord, Holly, R.D., and Rao, Linda, TOP SEED WITH ITS NUTRITIONAL POWERS: *Flax is the Next Nutritional Star,* Prevention Magazine, April 1997.

McIlwain, H., *Biochemistry and the Central Nervous System,* Boston, Little, Brown, 1959.

Pettegrew, J.W., Klunk, W.E., Panchalingam, K., et al, *Clinical and neurochemical effect of acetyl-L-carnitine treatment of mental decline in the elderly,* Drugs Exp Clin Res, 1994, 20:169-76.

Ramazanov, Dr. Zakir, Suarez, Dr. Maria del Mar Bernal; *Stress and Weight Management Using Rhodiola Rosea and Rhododendron Caucasicum,* Safe Goods, 1999.

Ressel, Dr. Ogi., *KIDS FIRST: Health with no Interference*, East Canaan, CT, New Century Publishing 2000, 2001.

Roberts, H.J., *Defense Against Alzheimer's Disease*, Sunshine Sentinel Press, 800.814.9800.

Sano, M., Ernesto, C., Thomas, R.G., et al, *A controlled trial of selegiline alpha-tocopherol or both as treatment for Alzheimer's*, New England Journal of Medicine, 1997, 336:1216-22.

Schmidt, Michael A., *SMART FATS: How dietary fats and oils affect mental, physical and emotional intelligence*, Berkeley, CA, Frog, Ltd., North Atlantic Books, 1997.

Schmidt, R., Hayn, M., Reinhart, B., et al, *PLASMA ANTIOXIDANTS AND COGNITIVE PERFORMANCE IN MIDDLE AGED AND OLDER ADULTS: Results of the Austrian Stroke Prevention Study*, Journal of the American Geriatric Society, 1998, 46:1407-10.

Simopoulos, M.D., Artemis, P., Robinson, Jo, *THE OMEGA PLAN: The Medically Proven Diet that Gives You the Essential Nutritional Balance*, New York, NY, Harper Collins Publishing, 1998.

Swartwout, Glen, *Electromagnetic Pollution Solutions*, AERI Publishing, Hilo, HI, 1991.

Whitaker, Dr. Julian M., *THE MEMORY SOLUTION: Dr. Julian Whitaker's 10-Step Program to Optimize Your Memory and Brain Function*, with Peggy Dance, Garden City Park, NY, Avery Publishing Group, 1999.

Wise, Sabina, *The Sugar Addict's Diet*, New Century Publishing 2000, March 2001.

West, David, Parker, Steve, *Brain Surgery for Beginners*, The Millbrook Press, Brookfield, CT, 1995.

Bibliography

From Safe Goods/New Century Publishing 2000

To order contact:
877.742.7078 toll free
905.471.5711

Other Books

A Doctor in Your Suitcase $7.95 US
Natural medicine for self-care   11.95 CA
when you are away from home.

The Brain Train $4.95 US
How to keep our brain healthy and wise.   7.95 CA
(Easy-to-read for school age children)

Cancer Disarmed $4.95 US
How cancer works and what can disarm it.   7.95 CA

The Fitness for Golfers Handbook $14.95 US
Taking your golf game to the next level.   19.95 CA

Kid's–First: Health with No Interference $12.95 US
Underlying causes and natural solutions for   19.95 CA
many of our children's most common illnesses.

Nutritional Leverage for Great Golf $9.95 US
How to improve your score on the back nine.   14.95 CA

Self-Care Anywhere $19.95 US
Powerful natural remedies   29.95 CA
for common health ailments.

Velvet Antler $9.95 US
Nature's superior tonic   14.95 CA

Index

Notes